This caregiver's journal belongs to:

_____

_____

_____

Contact details:

_____

_____

_____

_____

Activity & Caregiving Notes for _____ Date:_____

TOILETING

TIME							
U							
BM							

TIMES UP DURING THE NIGHT

_____   _____   _____   _____   _____

TODAY I HAD A SHOWER/WASHED MY HAIR/SPONGE BATH

Breakfast	
AM Snack	
Lunch	
PM Snack	
Dinner	
Drinks	

ACTIVITIES & OTHER COMMENTS

_____
_____
_____
_____
_____
_____

APPOINTMENTS: _____

HEALTH CONCERNS: _____

PLANS FOR TOMORROW:_____

PAIN LEVEL: _____HAPPINESS LEVEL:_____ALERTNESS LEVEL: _____

SUPPLIES NEEDED SOON:_____

MEDICATION TAKEN:_____

NOTES

_____
_____
_____

Activity & Caregiving Notes for _____ Date:_____

TOILETING

TIME							
U							
BM							

TIMES UP DURING THE NIGHT

_____   _____   _____   _____   _____

TODAY I HAD A SHOWER/WASHED MY HAIR/SPONGE BATH

Breakfast	
AM Snack	
Lunch	
PM Snack	
Dinner	
Drinks	

ACTIVITIES & OTHER COMMENTS

_____
_____
_____
_____
_____
_____

APPOINTMENTS: _____
HEALTH CONCERNS: _____
PLANS FOR TOMORROW: _____
PAIN LEVEL: _____HAPPINESS LEVEL:_____ALERTNESS LEVEL: _____
SUPPLIES NEEDED SOON: _____
MEDICATION TAKEN:_____

NOTES

_____
_____
_____

Activity & Caregiving Notes for _____ Date:_____

TOILETING

TIME							
U							
BM							

TIMES UP DURING THE NIGHT

_____ _____ _____ _____ _____

TODAY I HAD A SHOWER/WASHED MY HAIR/SPONGE BATH

Breakfast	
AM Snack	
Lunch	
PM Snack	
Dinner	
Drinks	

ACTIVITIES & OTHER COMMENTS

_____
_____
_____
_____
_____
_____

APPOINTMENTS: _____

HEALTH CONCERNS: _____

PLANS FOR TOMORROW: _____

PAIN LEVEL: _____ HAPPINESS LEVEL: _____ ALERTNESS LEVEL: _____

SUPPLIES NEEDED SOON: _____

MEDICATION TAKEN: _____

NOTES

_____
_____
_____

Activity & Caregiving Notes for _____ Date:_____

TOILETING

TIME							
U							
BM							

TIMES UP DURING THE NIGHT

_____   _____   _____   _____   _____

TODAY I HAD A SHOWER/WASHED MY HAIR/SPONGE BATH

Breakfast	
AM Snack	
Lunch	
PM Snack	
Dinner	
Drinks	

ACTIVITIES & OTHER COMMENTS

_____
_____
_____
_____
_____
_____

APPOINTMENTS: _____
HEALTH CONCERNS: _____
PLANS FOR TOMORROW: _____
PAIN LEVEL: _____HAPPINESS LEVEL:_____ALERTNESS LEVEL: _____
SUPPLIES NEEDED SOON:_____
MEDICATION TAKEN:_____

NOTES

_____
_____
_____

Activity & Caregiving Notes for _____ Date:_____

TOILETING

TIME								
U								
BM								

TIMES UP DURING THE NIGHT

_____ _____ _____ _____ _____

TODAY I HAD A SHOWER/WASHED MY HAIR/SPONGE BATH

Breakfast	
AM Snack	
Lunch	
PM Snack	
Dinner	
Drinks	

ACTIVITIES & OTHER COMMENTS

_____
_____
_____
_____
_____
_____

APPOINTMENTS: _____

HEALTH CONCERNS: _____

PLANS FOR TOMORROW: _____

PAIN LEVEL: _____ HAPPINESS LEVEL:_____ ALERTNESS LEVEL: _____

SUPPLIES NEEDED SOON: _____

MEDICATION TAKEN: _____

NOTES

_____
_____
_____

Activity & Caregiving Notes for _____ Date:_____

TOILETING

TIME							
U							
BM							

TIMES UP DURING THE NIGHT

_____   _____   _____   _____   _____

TODAY I HAD A SHOWER/WASHED MY HAIR/SPONGE BATH

Breakfast	
AM Snack	
Lunch	
PM Snack	
Dinner	
Drinks	

ACTIVITIES & OTHER COMMENTS

_____
_____
_____
_____
_____
_____

APPOINTMENTS: _____

HEALTH CONCERNS: _____

PLANS FOR TOMORROW:_____

PAIN LEVEL: _____HAPPINESS LEVEL:_____ALERTNESS LEVEL: _____

SUPPLIES NEEDED SOON:_____

MEDICATION TAKEN:_____

NOTES

_____
_____
_____

Activity & Caregiving Notes for _____ Date:_____

TOILETING

TIME							
U							
BM							

TIMES UP DURING THE NIGHT

_____ _____ _____ _____ _____

TODAY I HAD A SHOWER/WASHED MY HAIR/SPONGE BATH

Breakfast	
AM Snack	
Lunch	
PM Snack	
Dinner	
Drinks	

ACTIVITIES & OTHER COMMENTS

_____
_____
_____
_____
_____
_____

APPOINTMENTS: _____
HEALTH CONCERNS: _____
PLANS FOR TOMORROW: _____
PAIN LEVEL: _____ HAPPINESS LEVEL:_____ ALERTNESS LEVEL: _____
SUPPLIES NEEDED SOON:_____
MEDICATION TAKEN:_____

NOTES

_____
_____
_____

Activity & Caregiving Notes for _____ Date:_____

TOILETING

TIME							
U							
BM							

TIMES UP DURING THE NIGHT

_____ _____ _____ _____ _____

TODAY I HAD A SHOWER/WASHED MY HAIR/SPONGE BATH

Breakfast	
AM Snack	
Lunch	
PM Snack	
Dinner	
Drinks	

ACTIVITIES & OTHER COMMENTS

_____
_____
_____
_____
_____
_____

APPOINTMENTS: _____

HEALTH CONCERNS: _____

PLANS FOR TOMORROW: _____

PAIN LEVEL: _____HAPPINESS LEVEL:_____ALERTNESS LEVEL: _____

SUPPLIES NEEDED SOON:_____

MEDICATION TAKEN:_____

NOTES

_____
_____
_____

Activity & Caregiving Notes for _____ Date:_____

TOILETING

TIME							
U							
BM							

TIMES UP DURING THE NIGHT

_____ _____ _____ _____ _____

TODAY I HAD A SHOWER/WASHED MY HAIR/SPONGE BATH

Breakfast	
AM Snack	
Lunch	
PM Snack	
Dinner	
Drinks	

ACTIVITIES & OTHER COMMENTS

_____
_____
_____
_____
_____
_____

APPOINTMENTS: _____
HEALTH CONCERNS: _____
PLANS FOR TOMORROW: _____
PAIN LEVEL: _____HAPPINESS LEVEL:_____ALERTNESS LEVEL: _____
SUPPLIES NEEDED SOON:_____
MEDICATION TAKEN:_____

NOTES

_____
_____
_____

Activity & Caregiving Notes for _____ Date:_____

TOILETING

TIME							
U							
BM							

TIMES UP DURING THE NIGHT

_____   _____   _____   _____   _____

TODAY I HAD A SHOWER/WASHED MY HAIR/SPONGE BATH

Breakfast	
AM Snack	
Lunch	
PM Snack	
Dinner	
Drinks	

ACTIVITIES & OTHER COMMENTS

_____

_____

_____

_____

_____

_____

APPOINTMENTS: _____

HEALTH CONCERNS: _____

PLANS FOR TOMORROW: _____

PAIN LEVEL: _____HAPPINESS LEVEL:_____ALERTNESS LEVEL: _____

SUPPLIES NEEDED SOON:_____

MEDICATION TAKEN:_____

NOTES

_____

_____

_____

Activity & Caregiving Notes for _____ Date:_____

TOILETING

TIME								
U								
BM								

TIMES UP DURING THE NIGHT

_____   _____   _____   _____   _____

TODAY I HAD A SHOWER/WASHED MY HAIR/SPONGE BATH

Breakfast	
AM Snack	
Lunch	
PM Snack	
Dinner	
Drinks	

ACTIVITIES & OTHER COMMENTS

_____

_____

_____

_____

_____

_____

APPOINTMENTS: _____

HEALTH CONCERNS: _____

PLANS FOR TOMORROW: _____

PAIN LEVEL: _____ HAPPINESS LEVEL:_____ ALERTNESS LEVEL: _____

SUPPLIES NEEDED SOON: _____

MEDICATION TAKEN: _____

NOTES

_____

_____

_____

Activity & Caregiving Notes for _____ Date:_____

TOILETING

TIME							
U							
BM							

TIMES UP DURING THE NIGHT

_____   _____   _____   _____   _____

TODAY I HAD A SHOWER/WASHED MY HAIR/SPONGE BATH

Breakfast	
AM Snack	
Lunch	
PM Snack	
Dinner	
Drinks	

ACTIVITIES & OTHER COMMENTS

_____
_____
_____
_____
_____
_____

APPOINTMENTS: _____
HEALTH CONCERNS: _____
PLANS FOR TOMORROW: _____
PAIN LEVEL: _____HAPPINESS LEVEL:_____ALERTNESS LEVEL: _____
SUPPLIES NEEDED SOON: _____
MEDICATION TAKEN:_____

NOTES

_____
_____
_____

Activity & Caregiving Notes for _____ Date:_____

TOILETING

TIME							
U							
BM							

TIMES UP DURING THE NIGHT

_____   _____   _____   _____   _____

TODAY I HAD A SHOWER/WASHED MY HAIR/SPONGE BATH

Breakfast	
AM Snack	
Lunch	
PM Snack	
Dinner	
Drinks	

ACTIVITIES & OTHER COMMENTS

_____
_____
_____
_____
_____
_____

APPOINTMENTS: _____

HEALTH CONCERNS: _____

PLANS FOR TOMORROW: _____

PAIN LEVEL: _____HAPPINESS LEVEL:_____ALERTNESS LEVEL: _____

SUPPLIES NEEDED SOON:_____

MEDICATION TAKEN:_____

NOTES

_____
_____
_____

Activity & Caregiving Notes for _____ Date:_____

TOILETING

TIME							
U							
BM							

TIMES UP DURING THE NIGHT

_____   _____   _____   _____   _____

TODAY I HAD A SHOWER/WASHED MY HAIR/SPONGE BATH

Breakfast	
AM Snack	
Lunch	
PM Snack	
Dinner	
Drinks	

ACTIVITIES & OTHER COMMENTS

_____
_____
_____
_____
_____
_____

APPOINTMENTS: _____
HEALTH CONCERNS: _____
PLANS FOR TOMORROW: _____
PAIN LEVEL: _____HAPPINESS LEVEL:_____ALERTNESS LEVEL: _____
SUPPLIES NEEDED SOON: _____
MEDICATION TAKEN:_____

NOTES

_____
_____
_____

Activity & Caregiving Notes for _____ Date:_____

TOILETING

TIME								
U								
BM								

TIMES UP DURING THE NIGHT

_____   _____   _____   _____   _____

TODAY I HAD A SHOWER/WASHED MY HAIR/SPONGE BATH

Breakfast	
AM Snack	
Lunch	
PM Snack	
Dinner	
Drinks	

ACTIVITIES & OTHER COMMENTS

_____

_____

_____

_____

_____

_____

APPOINTMENTS: _____

HEALTH CONCERNS: _____

PLANS FOR TOMORROW: _____

PAIN LEVEL: _____HAPPINESS LEVEL:_____ALERTNESS LEVEL: _____

SUPPLIES NEEDED SOON:_____

MEDICATION TAKEN:_____

NOTES

_____

_____

_____

Activity & Caregiving Notes for _____ Date:_____

TOILETING

TIME							
U							
BM							

TIMES UP DURING THE NIGHT

_____ _____ _____ _____ _____

TODAY I HAD A SHOWER/WASHED MY HAIR/SPONGE BATH

Breakfast	
AM Snack	
Lunch	
PM Snack	
Dinner	
Drinks	

ACTIVITIES & OTHER COMMENTS

_____

_____

_____

_____

_____

_____

APPOINTMENTS: _____

HEALTH CONCERNS: _____

PLANS FOR TOMORROW: _____

PAIN LEVEL: _____HAPPINESS LEVEL:_____ALERTNESS LEVEL: _____

SUPPLIES NEEDED SOON:_____

MEDICATION TAKEN:_____

NOTES

_____

_____

_____

Activity & Caregiving Notes for _____ Date:_____

TOILETING

TIME							
U							
BM							

TIMES UP DURING THE NIGHT

_____   _____   _____   _____   _____

TODAY I HAD A SHOWER/WASHED MY HAIR/SPONGE BATH

Breakfast	
AM Snack	
Lunch	
PM Snack	
Dinner	
Drinks	

ACTIVITIES & OTHER COMMENTS

_____
_____
_____
_____
_____
_____

APPOINTMENTS: _____
HEALTH CONCERNS: _____
PLANS FOR TOMORROW: _____
PAIN LEVEL: _____HAPPINESS LEVEL:_____ALERTNESS LEVEL: _____
SUPPLIES NEEDED SOON: _____
MEDICATION TAKEN:_____

NOTES

_____
_____
_____

Activity & Caregiving Notes for _____ Date:_____

TOILETING

TIME							
U							
BM							

TIMES UP DURING THE NIGHT

_____ _____ _____ _____ _____

TODAY I HAD A SHOWER/WASHED MY HAIR/SPONGE BATH

Breakfast	
AM Snack	
Lunch	
PM Snack	
Dinner	
Drinks	

ACTIVITIES & OTHER COMMENTS

_____
_____
_____
_____
_____
_____

APPOINTMENTS: _____
HEALTH CONCERNS: _____
PLANS FOR TOMORROW:_____
PAIN LEVEL: _____HAPPINESS LEVEL:_____ALERTNESS LEVEL: _____
SUPPLIES NEEDED SOON:_____
MEDICATION TAKEN:_____

NOTES

_____
_____
_____

Activity & Caregiving Notes for _____ Date:_____

TOILETING

TIME							
U							
BM							

TIMES UP DURING THE NIGHT

_____ _____ _____ _____ _____

TODAY I HAD A SHOWER/WASHED MY HAIR/SPONGE BATH

Breakfast	
AM Snack	
Lunch	
PM Snack	
Dinner	
Drinks	

ACTIVITIES & OTHER COMMENTS

_____
_____
_____
_____
_____
_____

APPOINTMENTS: _____
HEALTH CONCERNS: _____
PLANS FOR TOMORROW:_____
PAIN LEVEL: _____HAPPINESS LEVEL:_____ALERTNESS LEVEL: _____
SUPPLIES NEEDED SOON:_____
MEDICATION TAKEN:_____

NOTES

_____
_____
_____

Activity & Caregiving Notes for _____ Date:_____

TOILETING

TIME							
U							
BM							

TIMES UP DURING THE NIGHT

_____ _____ _____ _____ _____

TODAY I HAD A SHOWER/WASHED MY HAIR/SPONGE BATH

Breakfast	
AM Snack	
Lunch	
PM Snack	
Dinner	
Drinks	

ACTIVITIES & OTHER COMMENTS

_____
_____
_____
_____
_____
_____

APPOINTMENTS: _____
HEALTH CONCERNS: _____
PLANS FOR TOMORROW: _____
PAIN LEVEL: _____HAPPINESS LEVEL:_____ALERTNESS LEVEL: _____
SUPPLIES NEEDED SOON:_____
MEDICATION TAKEN:_____

NOTES

_____
_____
_____

Activity & Caregiving Notes for _____ Date:_____

TOILETING

TIME							
U							
BM							

TIMES UP DURING THE NIGHT

_____   _____   _____   _____   _____

TODAY I HAD A SHOWER/WASHED MY HAIR/SPONGE BATH

Breakfast	
AM Snack	
Lunch	
PM Snack	
Dinner	
Drinks	

ACTIVITIES & OTHER COMMENTS

_____

_____

_____

_____

_____

_____

APPOINTMENTS: _____

HEALTH CONCERNS: _____

PLANS FOR TOMORROW: _____

PAIN LEVEL: _____ HAPPINESS LEVEL:_____ALERTNESS LEVEL: _____

SUPPLIES NEEDED SOON:_____

MEDICATION TAKEN:_____

NOTES

_____

_____

_____

Activity & Caregiving Notes for _____ Date:_____

TOILETING

TIME							
U							
BM							

TIMES UP DURING THE NIGHT

_____   _____   _____   _____   _____

TODAY I HAD A SHOWER/WASHED MY HAIR/SPONGE BATH

Breakfast	
AM Snack	
Lunch	
PM Snack	
Dinner	
Drinks	

ACTIVITIES & OTHER COMMENTS

_____

_____

_____

_____

_____

_____

APPOINTMENTS: _____

HEALTH CONCERNS: _____

PLANS FOR TOMORROW: _____

PAIN LEVEL: _____HAPPINESS LEVEL:_____ALERTNESS LEVEL: _____

SUPPLIES NEEDED SOON: _____

MEDICATION TAKEN:_____

NOTES

_____

_____

_____

Activity & Caregiving Notes for _____ Date:_____

TOILETING

TIME							
U							
BM							

TIMES UP DURING THE NIGHT

_____   _____   _____   _____   _____

TODAY I HAD A SHOWER/WASHED MY HAIR/SPONGE BATH

Breakfast	
AM Snack	
Lunch	
PM Snack	
Dinner	
Drinks	

ACTIVITIES & OTHER COMMENTS

_____

_____

_____

_____

_____

_____

APPOINTMENTS: _____

HEALTH CONCERNS: _____

PLANS FOR TOMORROW: _____

PAIN LEVEL: _____ HAPPINESS LEVEL: _____ ALERTNESS LEVEL: _____

SUPPLIES NEEDED SOON: _____

MEDICATION TAKEN: _____

NOTES

_____

_____

_____

Activity & Caregiving Notes for _____ Date:_____

TOILETING

TIME							
U							
BM							

TIMES UP DURING THE NIGHT

_____   _____   _____   _____   _____

TODAY I HAD A SHOWER/WASHED MY HAIR/SPONGE BATH

Breakfast	
AM Snack	
Lunch	
PM Snack	
Dinner	
Drinks	

ACTIVITIES & OTHER COMMENTS

_____
_____
_____
_____
_____
_____

APPOINTMENTS: _____
HEALTH CONCERNS: _____
PLANS FOR TOMORROW: _____
PAIN LEVEL: _____HAPPINESS LEVEL:_____ALERTNESS LEVEL: _____
SUPPLIES NEEDED SOON: _____
MEDICATION TAKEN:_____

NOTES

_____
_____
_____

Activity & Caregiving Notes for _____ Date:_____

TOILETING

TIME							
U							
BM							

TIMES UP DURING THE NIGHT

_____   _____   _____   _____   _____

TODAY I HAD A SHOWER/WASHED MY HAIR/SPONGE BATH

Breakfast	
AM Snack	
Lunch	
PM Snack	
Dinner	
Drinks	

ACTIVITIES & OTHER COMMENTS

_____
_____
_____
_____
_____
_____

APPOINTMENTS: _____
HEALTH CONCERNS: _____
PLANS FOR TOMORROW: _____
PAIN LEVEL: _____HAPPINESS LEVEL:_____ALERTNESS LEVEL: _____
SUPPLIES NEEDED SOON:_____
MEDICATION TAKEN:_____

NOTES

_____
_____
_____

Activity & Caregiving Notes for _____ Date:_____

TOILETING

TIME							
U							
BM							

TIMES UP DURING THE NIGHT

_____ _____ _____ _____ _____

TODAY I HAD A SHOWER/WASHED MY HAIR/SPONGE BATH

Breakfast	
AM Snack	
Lunch	
PM Snack	
Dinner	
Drinks	

ACTIVITIES & OTHER COMMENTS

_____
_____
_____
_____
_____
_____

APPOINTMENTS: _____

HEALTH CONCERNS: _____

PLANS FOR TOMORROW:_____

PAIN LEVEL: _____HAPPINESS LEVEL:_____ALERTNESS LEVEL: _____

SUPPLIES NEEDED SOON:_____

MEDICATION TAKEN:_____

NOTES

_____
_____
_____

Activity & Caregiving Notes for _____ Date:_____

TOILETING

TIME							
U							
BM							

TIMES UP DURING THE NIGHT

_____   _____   _____   _____   _____

TODAY I HAD A SHOWER/WASHED MY HAIR/SPONGE BATH

Breakfast	
AM Snack	
Lunch	
PM Snack	
Dinner	
Drinks	

ACTIVITIES & OTHER COMMENTS

_____

_____

_____

_____

_____

_____

APPOINTMENTS: _____

HEALTH CONCERNS: _____

PLANS FOR TOMORROW: _____

PAIN LEVEL: _____ HAPPINESS LEVEL:_____ ALERTNESS LEVEL: _____

SUPPLIES NEEDED SOON:_____

MEDICATION TAKEN:_____

NOTES

_____

_____

_____

Activity & Caregiving Notes for _____ Date:_____

TOILETING

TIME							
U							
BM							

TIMES UP DURING THE NIGHT

_____   _____   _____   _____   _____

TODAY I HAD A SHOWER/WASHED MY HAIR/SPONGE BATH

Breakfast	
AM Snack	
Lunch	
PM Snack	
Dinner	
Drinks	

ACTIVITIES & OTHER COMMENTS

_____

_____

_____

_____

_____

_____

APPOINTMENTS: _____

HEALTH CONCERNS: _____

PLANS FOR TOMORROW: _____

PAIN LEVEL: _____ HAPPINESS LEVEL:_____ ALERTNESS LEVEL: _____

SUPPLIES NEEDED SOON:_____

MEDICATION TAKEN:_____

NOTES

_____

_____

_____

Activity & Caregiving Notes for _____ Date:_____

TOILETING

TIME								
U								
BM								

TIMES UP DURING THE NIGHT

_____ _____ _____ _____ _____

TODAY I HAD A SHOWER/WASHED MY HAIR/SPONGE BATH

Breakfast	
AM Snack	
Lunch	
PM Snack	
Dinner	
Drinks	

ACTIVITIES & OTHER COMMENTS

_____
_____
_____
_____
_____
_____

APPOINTMENTS: _____

HEALTH CONCERNS: _____

PLANS FOR TOMORROW:_____

PAIN LEVEL: _____HAPPINESS LEVEL:_____ALERTNESS LEVEL: _____

SUPPLIES NEEDED SOON:_____

MEDICATION TAKEN:_____

NOTES

_____
_____
_____

Activity & Caregiving Notes for _____ Date:_____

TOILETING

TIME							
U							
BM							

TIMES UP DURING THE NIGHT

_____   _____   _____   _____   _____

TODAY I HAD A SHOWER/WASHED MY HAIR/SPONGE BATH

Breakfast	
AM Snack	
Lunch	
PM Snack	
Dinner	
Drinks	

ACTIVITIES & OTHER COMMENTS

_____
_____
_____
_____
_____
_____

APPOINTMENTS: _____

HEALTH CONCERNS: _____

PLANS FOR TOMORROW: _____

PAIN LEVEL: _____ HAPPINESS LEVEL:_____ ALERTNESS LEVEL: _____

SUPPLIES NEEDED SOON: _____

MEDICATION TAKEN:_____

NOTES

_____
_____
_____

Activity & Caregiving Notes for _____ Date:_____

TOILETING

TIME								
U								
BM								

TIMES UP DURING THE NIGHT

_____ _____ _____ _____ _____

TODAY I HAD A SHOWER/WASHED MY HAIR/SPONGE BATH

Breakfast	
AM Snack	
Lunch	
PM Snack	
Dinner	
Drinks	

ACTIVITIES & OTHER COMMENTS

_____
_____
_____
_____
_____
_____

APPOINTMENTS: _____
HEALTH CONCERNS: _____
PLANS FOR TOMORROW:_____
PAIN LEVEL: _____HAPPINESS LEVEL:_____ALERTNESS LEVEL: _____
SUPPLIES NEEDED SOON:_____
MEDICATION TAKEN:_____

NOTES

_____
_____
_____

Activity & Caregiving Notes for _____ Date:_____

TOILETING

TIME							
U							
BM							

TIMES UP DURING THE NIGHT

_____   _____   _____   _____   _____

TODAY I HAD A SHOWER/WASHED MY HAIR/SPONGE BATH

Breakfast	
AM Snack	
Lunch	
PM Snack	
Dinner	
Drinks	

ACTIVITIES & OTHER COMMENTS

_____
_____
_____
_____
_____
_____
_____

APPOINTMENTS: _____

HEALTH CONCERNS: _____

PLANS FOR TOMORROW: _____

PAIN LEVEL: _____HAPPINESS LEVEL:_____ALERTNESS LEVEL: _____

SUPPLIES NEEDED SOON:_____

MEDICATION TAKEN:_____

NOTES

_____
_____
_____

Activity & Caregiving Notes for _____ Date:_____

TOILETING

TIME							
U							
BM							

TIMES UP DURING THE NIGHT

_____ _____ _____ _____ _____

TODAY I HAD A SHOWER/WASHED MY HAIR/SPONGE BATH

Breakfast	
AM Snack	
Lunch	
PM Snack	
Dinner	
Drinks	

ACTIVITIES & OTHER COMMENTS

_____
_____
_____
_____
_____
_____

APPOINTMENTS: _____

HEALTH CONCERNS: _____

PLANS FOR TOMORROW: _____

PAIN LEVEL: _____ HAPPINESS LEVEL:_____ALERTNESS LEVEL: _____

SUPPLIES NEEDED SOON:_____

MEDICATION TAKEN:_____

NOTES

_____
_____
_____

Activity & Caregiving Notes for _____ Date:_____

TOILETING

TIME							
U							
BM							

TIMES UP DURING THE NIGHT

_____ _____ _____ _____ _____

TODAY I HAD A SHOWER/WASHED MY HAIR/SPONGE BATH

Breakfast	
AM Snack	
Lunch	
PM Snack	
Dinner	
Drinks	

ACTIVITIES & OTHER COMMENTS

_____
_____
_____
_____
_____
_____

APPOINTMENTS: _____

HEALTH CONCERNS: _____

PLANS FOR TOMORROW: _____

PAIN LEVEL: _____HAPPINESS LEVEL:_____ALERTNESS LEVEL: _____

SUPPLIES NEEDED SOON:_____

MEDICATION TAKEN:_____

NOTES

_____
_____
_____

Activity & Caregiving Notes for _____ Date:_____

TOILETING

TIME							
U							
BM							

TIMES UP DURING THE NIGHT

_____   _____   _____   _____   _____

TODAY I HAD A SHOWER/WASHED MY HAIR/SPONGE BATH

Breakfast	
AM Snack	
Lunch	
PM Snack	
Dinner	
Drinks	

ACTIVITIES & OTHER COMMENTS

_____

_____

_____

_____

_____

_____

APPOINTMENTS: _____

HEALTH CONCERNS: _____

PLANS FOR TOMORROW: _____

PAIN LEVEL: _____HAPPINESS LEVEL:_____ALERTNESS LEVEL: _____

SUPPLIES NEEDED SOON: _____

MEDICATION TAKEN:_____

NOTES

_____

_____

_____

Activity & Caregiving Notes for _____ Date:_____

TOILETING

TIME							
U							
BM							

TIMES UP DURING THE NIGHT

_____ _____ _____ _____ _____

TODAY I HAD A SHOWER/WASHED MY HAIR/SPONGE BATH

Breakfast	
AM Snack	
Lunch	
PM Snack	
Dinner	
Drinks	

ACTIVITIES & OTHER COMMENTS

_____
_____
_____
_____
_____
_____

APPOINTMENTS: _____

HEALTH CONCERNS: _____

PLANS FOR TOMORROW: _____

PAIN LEVEL: _____HAPPINESS LEVEL:_____ALERTNESS LEVEL: _____

SUPPLIES NEEDED SOON: _____

MEDICATION TAKEN: _____

NOTES

_____
_____
_____

Activity & Caregiving Notes for _____ Date:_____

TOILETING

TIME							
U							
BM							

TIMES UP DURING THE NIGHT

_____ _____ _____ _____ _____

TODAY I HAD A SHOWER/WASHED MY HAIR/SPONGE BATH

Breakfast	
AM Snack	
Lunch	
PM Snack	
Dinner	
Drinks	

ACTIVITIES & OTHER COMMENTS

_____
_____
_____
_____
_____
_____

APPOINTMENTS: _____
HEALTH CONCERNS: _____
PLANS FOR TOMORROW: _____
PAIN LEVEL: _____HAPPINESS LEVEL:_____ALERTNESS LEVEL: _____
SUPPLIES NEEDED SOON:_____
MEDICATION TAKEN:_____

NOTES

_____
_____
_____

Activity & Caregiving Notes for _____ Date:_____

TOILETING

TIME							
U							
BM							

TIMES UP DURING THE NIGHT

_____ _____ _____ _____ _____

TODAY I HAD A SHOWER/WASHED MY HAIR/SPONGE BATH

Breakfast	
AM Snack	
Lunch	
PM Snack	
Dinner	
Drinks	

ACTIVITIES & OTHER COMMENTS

_____
_____
_____
_____
_____
_____

APPOINTMENTS: _____
HEALTH CONCERNS: _____
PLANS FOR TOMORROW:_____
PAIN LEVEL: _____HAPPINESS LEVEL:_____ALERTNESS LEVEL: _____
SUPPLIES NEEDED SOON: _____
MEDICATION TAKEN:_____

NOTES

_____
_____
_____

Activity & Caregiving Notes for _____ Date:_____

TOILETING

TIME								
U								
BM								

TIMES UP DURING THE NIGHT

_____   _____   _____   _____   _____

TODAY I HAD A SHOWER/WASHED MY HAIR/SPONGE BATH

Breakfast	
AM Snack	
Lunch	
PM Snack	
Dinner	
Drinks	

ACTIVITIES & OTHER COMMENTS

_____
_____
_____
_____
_____
_____

APPOINTMENTS: _____
HEALTH CONCERNS: _____
PLANS FOR TOMORROW: _____
PAIN LEVEL: _____HAPPINESS LEVEL:_____ALERTNESS LEVEL: _____
SUPPLIES NEEDED SOON: _____
MEDICATION TAKEN:_____

NOTES

_____
_____
_____

Activity & Caregiving Notes for _____ Date:_____

TOILETING

TIME							
U							
BM							

TIMES UP DURING THE NIGHT

_____ _____ _____ _____ _____

TODAY I HAD A SHOWER/WASHED MY HAIR/SPONGE BATH

Breakfast	
AM Snack	
Lunch	
PM Snack	
Dinner	
Drinks	

ACTIVITIES & OTHER COMMENTS

_____
_____
_____
_____
_____
_____

APPOINTMENTS: _____
HEALTH CONCERNS: _____
PLANS FOR TOMORROW: _____
PAIN LEVEL: _____HAPPINESS LEVEL:_____ALERTNESS LEVEL: _____
SUPPLIES NEEDED SOON:_____
MEDICATION TAKEN:_____

NOTES

_____
_____
_____

Activity & Caregiving Notes for _____ Date:_____

TOILETING

TIME								
U								
BM								

TIMES UP DURING THE NIGHT

_____   _____   _____   _____   _____

TODAY I HAD A SHOWER/WASHED MY HAIR/SPONGE BATH

Breakfast	
AM Snack	
Lunch	
PM Snack	
Dinner	
Drinks	

ACTIVITIES & OTHER COMMENTS

_____
_____
_____
_____
_____
_____

APPOINTMENTS: _____
HEALTH CONCERNS: _____
PLANS FOR TOMORROW: _____
PAIN LEVEL: _____HAPPINESS LEVEL:_____ALERTNESS LEVEL: _____
SUPPLIES NEEDED SOON: _____
MEDICATION TAKEN: _____

NOTES

_____
_____
_____

Activity & Caregiving Notes for _____ Date:_____

TOILETING

TIME							
U							
BM							

TIMES UP DURING THE NIGHT

_____   _____   _____   _____   _____

TODAY I HAD A SHOWER/WASHED MY HAIR/SPONGE BATH

Breakfast	
AM Snack	
Lunch	
PM Snack	
Dinner	
Drinks	

ACTIVITIES & OTHER COMMENTS

_____
_____
_____
_____
_____
_____

APPOINTMENTS: _____

HEALTH CONCERNS: _____

PLANS FOR TOMORROW: _____

PAIN LEVEL: _____HAPPINESS LEVEL:_____ALERTNESS LEVEL: _____

SUPPLIES NEEDED SOON:_____

MEDICATION TAKEN:_____

NOTES

_____
_____
_____

Activity & Caregiving Notes for _____ Date:_____

TOILETING

TIME							
U							
BM							

TIMES UP DURING THE NIGHT

_____   _____   _____   _____   _____

TODAY I HAD A SHOWER/WASHED MY HAIR/SPONGE BATH

Breakfast	
AM Snack	
Lunch	
PM Snack	
Dinner	
Drinks	

ACTIVITIES & OTHER COMMENTS

_____

_____

_____

_____

_____

_____

APPOINTMENTS: _____

HEALTH CONCERNS: _____

PLANS FOR TOMORROW: _____

PAIN LEVEL: _____HAPPINESS LEVEL:_____ALERTNESS LEVEL: _____

SUPPLIES NEEDED SOON:_____

MEDICATION TAKEN:_____

NOTES

_____

_____

_____

Activity & Caregiving Notes for _____ Date:_____

TOILETING

TIME							
U							
BM							

TIMES UP DURING THE NIGHT

_____ _____ _____ _____ _____

TODAY I HAD A SHOWER/WASHED MY HAIR/SPONGE BATH

Breakfast	
AM Snack	
Lunch	
PM Snack	
Dinner	
Drinks	

ACTIVITIES & OTHER COMMENTS

_____
_____
_____
_____
_____
_____

APPOINTMENTS: _____
HEALTH CONCERNS: _____
PLANS FOR TOMORROW: _____
PAIN LEVEL: _____HAPPINESS LEVEL:_____ALERTNESS LEVEL: _____
SUPPLIES NEEDED SOON: _____
MEDICATION TAKEN:_____

NOTES

_____
_____
_____

Activity & Caregiving Notes for _____ Date:_____

TOILETING

TIME							
U							
BM							

TIMES UP DURING THE NIGHT

_____   _____   _____   _____   _____

TODAY I HAD A SHOWER/WASHED MY HAIR/SPONGE BATH

Breakfast	
AM Snack	
Lunch	
PM Snack	
Dinner	
Drinks	

ACTIVITIES & OTHER COMMENTS

_____

_____

_____

_____

_____

_____

APPOINTMENTS: _____

HEALTH CONCERNS: _____

PLANS FOR TOMORROW: _____

PAIN LEVEL: _____HAPPINESS LEVEL:_____ALERTNESS LEVEL: _____

SUPPLIES NEEDED SOON: _____

MEDICATION TAKEN: _____

NOTES

_____

_____

_____

Activity & Caregiving Notes for _____ Date:_____

TOILETING

TIME								
U								
BM								

TIMES UP DURING THE NIGHT

_____   _____   _____   _____   _____

TODAY I HAD A SHOWER/WASHED MY HAIR/SPONGE BATH

Breakfast	
AM Snack	
Lunch	
PM Snack	
Dinner	
Drinks	

ACTIVITIES & OTHER COMMENTS

_____
_____
_____
_____
_____
_____

APPOINTMENTS: _____

HEALTH CONCERNS: _____

PLANS FOR TOMORROW: _____

PAIN LEVEL: _____HAPPINESS LEVEL:_____ALERTNESS LEVEL: _____

SUPPLIES NEEDED SOON:_____

MEDICATION TAKEN:_____

NOTES

_____
_____
_____

Activity & Caregiving Notes for _____ Date:_____

TOILETING

TIME							
U							
BM							

TIMES UP DURING THE NIGHT

_____ _____ _____ _____ _____

TODAY I HAD A SHOWER/WASHED MY HAIR/SPONGE BATH

Breakfast	
AM Snack	
Lunch	
PM Snack	
Dinner	
Drinks	

ACTIVITIES & OTHER COMMENTS

_____
_____
_____
_____
_____
_____

APPOINTMENTS: _____

HEALTH CONCERNS: _____

PLANS FOR TOMORROW: _____

PAIN LEVEL: _____ HAPPINESS LEVEL: _____ ALERTNESS LEVEL: _____

SUPPLIES NEEDED SOON: _____

MEDICATION TAKEN: _____

NOTES

_____
_____
_____

Activity & Caregiving Notes for _____ Date:_____

TOILETING

TIME								
U								
BM								

TIMES UP DURING THE NIGHT

_____   _____   _____   _____   _____

TODAY I HAD A SHOWER/WASHED MY HAIR/SPONGE BATH

Breakfast	
AM Snack	
Lunch	
PM Snack	
Dinner	
Drinks	

ACTIVITIES & OTHER COMMENTS

_____
_____
_____
_____
_____
_____

APPOINTMENTS: _____
HEALTH CONCERNS: _____
PLANS FOR TOMORROW: _____
PAIN LEVEL: _____HAPPINESS LEVEL:_____ALERTNESS LEVEL: _____
SUPPLIES NEEDED SOON: _____
MEDICATION TAKEN:_____

NOTES

_____
_____
_____

Activity & Caregiving Notes for _____ Date:_____

TOILETING

TIME							
U							
BM							

TIMES UP DURING THE NIGHT

_____ _____ _____ _____ _____

TODAY I HAD A SHOWER/WASHED MY HAIR/SPONGE BATH

Breakfast	
AM Snack	
Lunch	
PM Snack	
Dinner	
Drinks	

ACTIVITIES & OTHER COMMENTS

_____
_____
_____
_____
_____
_____
_____

APPOINTMENTS: _____
HEALTH CONCERNS: _____
PLANS FOR TOMORROW: _____
PAIN LEVEL: _____HAPPINESS LEVEL:_____ALERTNESS LEVEL: _____
SUPPLIES NEEDED SOON: _____
MEDICATION TAKEN:_____

NOTES

_____
_____
_____

Activity & Caregiving Notes for _____ Date:_____

TOILETING

TIME							
U							
BM							

TIMES UP DURING THE NIGHT

_____   _____   _____   _____   _____

TODAY I HAD A SHOWER/WASHED MY HAIR/SPONGE BATH

Breakfast	
AM Snack	
Lunch	
PM Snack	
Dinner	
Drinks	

ACTIVITIES & OTHER COMMENTS

_____
_____
_____
_____
_____
_____

APPOINTMENTS: _____
HEALTH CONCERNS: _____
PLANS FOR TOMORROW: _____
PAIN LEVEL: _____HAPPINESS LEVEL:_____ALERTNESS LEVEL: _____
SUPPLIES NEEDED SOON:_____
MEDICATION TAKEN:_____

NOTES

_____
_____
_____

Activity & Caregiving Notes for _____ Date:_____

TOILETING

TIME							
U							
BM							

TIMES UP DURING THE NIGHT

_____   _____   _____   _____   _____

TODAY I HAD A SHOWER/WASHED MY HAIR/SPONGE BATH

Breakfast	
AM Snack	
Lunch	
PM Snack	
Dinner	
Drinks	

ACTIVITIES & OTHER COMMENTS

_____

_____

_____

_____

_____

_____

APPOINTMENTS: _____

HEALTH CONCERNS: _____

PLANS FOR TOMORROW:_____

PAIN LEVEL: _____HAPPINESS LEVEL:_____ALERTNESS LEVEL: _____

SUPPLIES NEEDED SOON:_____

MEDICATION TAKEN:_____

NOTES

_____

_____

_____

Activity & Caregiving Notes for _____ Date:_____

TOILETING

TIME							
U							
BM							

TIMES UP DURING THE NIGHT

_____   _____   _____   _____   _____

TODAY I HAD A SHOWER/WASHED MY HAIR/SPONGE BATH

Breakfast	
AM Snack	
Lunch	
PM Snack	
Dinner	
Drinks	

ACTIVITIES & OTHER COMMENTS

_____

_____

_____

_____

_____

_____

APPOINTMENTS: _____

HEALTH CONCERNS: _____

PLANS FOR TOMORROW: _____

PAIN LEVEL: _____HAPPINESS LEVEL:_____ALERTNESS LEVEL: _____

SUPPLIES NEEDED SOON:_____

MEDICATION TAKEN:_____

NOTES

_____

_____

_____

Activity & Caregiving Notes for _____ Date:_____

TOILETING

TIME							
U							
BM							

TIMES UP DURING THE NIGHT

_____   _____   _____   _____   _____

TODAY I HAD A SHOWER/WASHED MY HAIR/SPONGE BATH

Breakfast	
AM Snack	
Lunch	
PM Snack	
Dinner	
Drinks	

ACTIVITIES & OTHER COMMENTS

_____
_____
_____
_____
_____
_____

APPOINTMENTS: _____

HEALTH CONCERNS: _____

PLANS FOR TOMORROW: _____

PAIN LEVEL: _____HAPPINESS LEVEL:_____ALERTNESS LEVEL: _____

SUPPLIES NEEDED SOON: _____

MEDICATION TAKEN: _____

NOTES

_____
_____
_____

Activity & Caregiving Notes for _____ Date:_____

TOILETING

TIME							
U							
BM							

TIMES UP DURING THE NIGHT

_____ _____ _____ _____ _____

TODAY I HAD A SHOWER/WASHED MY HAIR/SPONGE BATH

Breakfast	
AM Snack	
Lunch	
PM Snack	
Dinner	
Drinks	

ACTIVITIES & OTHER COMMENTS

_____
_____
_____
_____
_____
_____

APPOINTMENTS: _____
HEALTH CONCERNS: _____
PLANS FOR TOMORROW:_____
PAIN LEVEL: _____HAPPINESS LEVEL:_____ALERTNESS LEVEL: _____
SUPPLIES NEEDED SOON: _____
MEDICATION TAKEN:_____

NOTES

_____
_____
_____

Activity & Caregiving Notes for _____ Date:_____

TOILETING

TIME							
U							
BM							

TIMES UP DURING THE NIGHT

_____   _____   _____   _____   _____

TODAY I HAD A SHOWER/WASHED MY HAIR/SPONGE BATH

Breakfast	
AM Snack	
Lunch	
PM Snack	
Dinner	
Drinks	

ACTIVITIES & OTHER COMMENTS

_____
_____
_____
_____
_____
_____

APPOINTMENTS: _____
HEALTH CONCERNS: _____
PLANS FOR TOMORROW: _____
PAIN LEVEL: _____HAPPINESS LEVEL:_____ALERTNESS LEVEL: _____
SUPPLIES NEEDED SOON:_____
MEDICATION TAKEN:_____

NOTES

_____
_____
_____

Activity & Caregiving Notes for _____ Date:_____

TOILETING

TIME							
U							
BM							

TIMES UP DURING THE NIGHT

_____   _____   _____   _____   _____

TODAY I HAD A SHOWER/WASHED MY HAIR/SPONGE BATH

Breakfast	
AM Snack	
Lunch	
PM Snack	
Dinner	
Drinks	

ACTIVITIES & OTHER COMMENTS

_____
_____
_____
_____
_____
_____

APPOINTMENTS: _____
HEALTH CONCERNS: _____
PLANS FOR TOMORROW: _____
PAIN LEVEL: _____HAPPINESS LEVEL:_____ALERTNESS LEVEL: _____
SUPPLIES NEEDED SOON:_____
MEDICATION TAKEN:_____

NOTES

_____
_____
_____

Activity & Caregiving Notes for _____ Date:_____

TOILETING

TIME								
U								
BM								

TIMES UP DURING THE NIGHT

_____ _____ _____ _____ _____

TODAY I HAD A SHOWER/WASHED MY HAIR/SPONGE BATH

Breakfast	
AM Snack	
Lunch	
PM Snack	
Dinner	
Drinks	

ACTIVITIES & OTHER COMMENTS

_____
_____
_____
_____
_____
_____

APPOINTMENTS: _____

HEALTH CONCERNS: _____

PLANS FOR TOMORROW:_____

PAIN LEVEL: _____HAPPINESS LEVEL:_____ALERTNESS LEVEL: _____

SUPPLIES NEEDED SOON:_____

MEDICATION TAKEN:_____

NOTES

_____
_____
_____

Activity & Caregiving Notes for _____ Date:_____

TOILETING

TIME							
U							
BM							

TIMES UP DURING THE NIGHT

_____   _____   _____   _____   _____

TODAY I HAD A SHOWER/WASHED MY HAIR/SPONGE BATH

Breakfast	
AM Snack	
Lunch	
PM Snack	
Dinner	
Drinks	

ACTIVITIES & OTHER COMMENTS

_____
_____
_____
_____
_____
_____

APPOINTMENTS: _____
HEALTH CONCERNS: _____
PLANS FOR TOMORROW: _____
PAIN LEVEL: _____HAPPINESS LEVEL:_____ALERTNESS LEVEL: _____
SUPPLIES NEEDED SOON:_____
MEDICATION TAKEN:_____

NOTES

_____
_____
_____

Activity & Caregiving Notes for _____ Date:_____

TOILETING

TIME								
U								
BM								

TIMES UP DURING THE NIGHT

_____   _____   _____   _____   _____

TODAY I HAD A SHOWER/WASHED MY HAIR/SPONGE BATH

Breakfast	
AM Snack	
Lunch	
PM Snack	
Dinner	
Drinks	

ACTIVITIES & OTHER COMMENTS

_____
_____
_____
_____
_____
_____

APPOINTMENTS: _____

HEALTH CONCERNS: _____

PLANS FOR TOMORROW: _____

PAIN LEVEL: _____ HAPPINESS LEVEL:_____ ALERTNESS LEVEL: _____

SUPPLIES NEEDED SOON: _____

MEDICATION TAKEN:_____

NOTES

_____
_____
_____

Activity & Caregiving Notes for _____ Date:_____

TOILETING

TIME							
U							
BM							

TIMES UP DURING THE NIGHT

_____   _____   _____   _____   _____

TODAY I HAD A SHOWER/WASHED MY HAIR/SPONGE BATH

Breakfast	
AM Snack	
Lunch	
PM Snack	
Dinner	
Drinks	

ACTIVITIES & OTHER COMMENTS

_____

_____

_____

_____

_____

_____

APPOINTMENTS: _____

HEALTH CONCERNS: _____

PLANS FOR TOMORROW: _____

PAIN LEVEL: _____HAPPINESS LEVEL:_____ALERTNESS LEVEL: _____

SUPPLIES NEEDED SOON:_____

MEDICATION TAKEN:_____

NOTES

_____

_____

_____

Activity & Caregiving Notes for _____ Date:_____

TOILETING

TIME							
U							
BM							

TIMES UP DURING THE NIGHT

_____   _____   _____   _____   _____

TODAY I HAD A SHOWER/WASHED MY HAIR/SPONGE BATH

Breakfast	
AM Snack	
Lunch	
PM Snack	
Dinner	
Drinks	

ACTIVITIES & OTHER COMMENTS

_____

_____

_____

_____

_____

_____

APPOINTMENTS: _____

HEALTH CONCERNS: _____

PLANS FOR TOMORROW: _____

PAIN LEVEL: _____HAPPINESS LEVEL:_____ALERTNESS LEVEL: _____

SUPPLIES NEEDED SOON:_____

MEDICATION TAKEN:_____

NOTES

_____

_____

_____

Activity & Caregiving Notes for _____ Date:_____

TOILETING

TIME							
U							
BM							

TIMES UP DURING THE NIGHT

_____   _____   _____   _____   _____

TODAY I HAD A SHOWER/WASHED MY HAIR/SPONGE BATH

Breakfast	
AM Snack	
Lunch	
PM Snack	
Dinner	
Drinks	

ACTIVITIES & OTHER COMMENTS

_____
_____
_____
_____
_____
_____

APPOINTMENTS: _____

HEALTH CONCERNS: _____

PLANS FOR TOMORROW: _____

PAIN LEVEL: _____HAPPINESS LEVEL:_____ALERTNESS LEVEL: _____

SUPPLIES NEEDED SOON: _____

MEDICATION TAKEN:_____

NOTES

_____
_____
_____

Activity & Caregiving Notes for _____ Date:_____

TOILETING

TIME							
U							
BM							

TIMES UP DURING THE NIGHT

_____   _____   _____   _____   _____

TODAY I HAD A SHOWER/WASHED MY HAIR/SPONGE BATH

Breakfast	
AM Snack	
Lunch	
PM Snack	
Dinner	
Drinks	

ACTIVITIES & OTHER COMMENTS

_____
_____
_____
_____
_____
_____

APPOINTMENTS: _____

HEALTH CONCERNS: _____

PLANS FOR TOMORROW: _____

PAIN LEVEL: _____ HAPPINESS LEVEL:_____ALERTNESS LEVEL: _____

SUPPLIES NEEDED SOON:_____

MEDICATION TAKEN:_____

NOTES

_____
_____
_____

Activity & Caregiving Notes for _____ Date:_____

TOILETING

TIME							
U							
BM							

TIMES UP DURING THE NIGHT

_____   _____   _____   _____   _____

TODAY I HAD A SHOWER/WASHED MY HAIR/SPONGE BATH

Breakfast	
AM Snack	
Lunch	
PM Snack	
Dinner	
Drinks	

ACTIVITIES & OTHER COMMENTS

_____
_____
_____
_____
_____
_____

APPOINTMENTS: _____
HEALTH CONCERNS: _____
PLANS FOR TOMORROW: _____
PAIN LEVEL: _____HAPPINESS LEVEL:_____ALERTNESS LEVEL: _____
SUPPLIES NEEDED SOON: _____
MEDICATION TAKEN:_____

NOTES

_____
_____
_____

Activity & Caregiving Notes for _____ Date:_____

TOILETING

TIME							
U							
BM							

TIMES UP DURING THE NIGHT

_____   _____   _____   _____   _____

TODAY I HAD A SHOWER/WASHED MY HAIR/SPONGE BATH

Breakfast	
AM Snack	
Lunch	
PM Snack	
Dinner	
Drinks	

ACTIVITIES & OTHER COMMENTS

_____

_____

_____

_____

_____

_____

APPOINTMENTS: _____

HEALTH CONCERNS: _____

PLANS FOR TOMORROW: _____

PAIN LEVEL: _____ HAPPINESS LEVEL:_____ ALERTNESS LEVEL: _____

SUPPLIES NEEDED SOON:_____

MEDICATION TAKEN:_____

NOTES

_____

_____

_____

Activity & Caregiving Notes for _____ Date:_____

TOILETING

TIME							
U							
BM							

TIMES UP DURING THE NIGHT

_____   _____   _____   _____   _____

TODAY I HAD A SHOWER/WASHED MY HAIR/SPONGE BATH

Breakfast	
AM Snack	
Lunch	
PM Snack	
Dinner	
Drinks	

ACTIVITIES & OTHER COMMENTS

_____
_____
_____
_____
_____
_____

APPOINTMENTS: _____

HEALTH CONCERNS: _____

PLANS FOR TOMORROW: _____

PAIN LEVEL: _____HAPPINESS LEVEL:_____ALERTNESS LEVEL: _____

SUPPLIES NEEDED SOON:_____

MEDICATION TAKEN:_____

NOTES

_____
_____
_____

Activity & Caregiving Notes for _____ Date:_____

TOILETING

TIME							
U							
BM							

TIMES UP DURING THE NIGHT

_____   _____   _____   _____   _____

TODAY I HAD A SHOWER/WASHED MY HAIR/SPONGE BATH

Breakfast	
AM Snack	
Lunch	
PM Snack	
Dinner	
Drinks	

ACTIVITIES & OTHER COMMENTS

_____

_____

_____

_____

_____

_____

APPOINTMENTS: _____

HEALTH CONCERNS: _____

PLANS FOR TOMORROW: _____

PAIN LEVEL: _____HAPPINESS LEVEL:_____ALERTNESS LEVEL: _____

SUPPLIES NEEDED SOON:_____

MEDICATION TAKEN:_____

NOTES

_____

_____

_____

Activity & Caregiving Notes for _____ Date:_____

TOILETING

TIME							
U							
BM							

TIMES UP DURING THE NIGHT

_____ _____ _____ _____ _____

TODAY I HAD A SHOWER/WASHED MY HAIR/SPONGE BATH

Breakfast	
AM Snack	
Lunch	
PM Snack	
Dinner	
Drinks	

ACTIVITIES & OTHER COMMENTS

_____
_____
_____
_____
_____
_____

APPOINTMENTS: _____

HEALTH CONCERNS: _____

PLANS FOR TOMORROW: _____

PAIN LEVEL: _____ HAPPINESS LEVEL:_____ ALERTNESS LEVEL: _____

SUPPLIES NEEDED SOON:_____

MEDICATION TAKEN:_____

NOTES

_____
_____
_____

Activity & Caregiving Notes for _____ Date:_____

TOILETING

TIME							
U							
BM							

TIMES UP DURING THE NIGHT

_____ _____ _____ _____ _____

TODAY I HAD A SHOWER/WASHED MY HAIR/SPONGE BATH

Breakfast	
AM Snack	
Lunch	
PM Snack	
Dinner	
Drinks	

ACTIVITIES & OTHER COMMENTS

_____

_____

_____

_____

_____

_____

APPOINTMENTS: _____

HEALTH CONCERNS: _____

PLANS FOR TOMORROW:_____

PAIN LEVEL: _____HAPPINESS LEVEL:_____ALERTNESS LEVEL: _____

SUPPLIES NEEDED SOON:_____

MEDICATION TAKEN:_____

NOTES

_____

_____

_____

Activity & Caregiving Notes for _____ Date:_____

TOILETING

TIME							
U							
BM							

TIMES UP DURING THE NIGHT

_____   _____   _____   _____   _____

TODAY I HAD A SHOWER/WASHED MY HAIR/SPONGE BATH

Breakfast	
AM Snack	
Lunch	
PM Snack	
Dinner	
Drinks	

ACTIVITIES & OTHER COMMENTS

_____
_____
_____
_____
_____
_____

APPOINTMENTS: _____

HEALTH CONCERNS: _____

PLANS FOR TOMORROW: _____

PAIN LEVEL: _____HAPPINESS LEVEL:_____ALERTNESS LEVEL: _____

SUPPLIES NEEDED SOON: _____

MEDICATION TAKEN:_____

NOTES

_____
_____
_____

Activity & Caregiving Notes for _____ Date:_____

TOILETING

TIME							
U							
BM							

TIMES UP DURING THE NIGHT

_____   _____   _____   _____   _____

TODAY I HAD A SHOWER/WASHED MY HAIR/SPONGE BATH

Breakfast	
AM Snack	
Lunch	
PM Snack	
Dinner	
Drinks	

ACTIVITIES & OTHER COMMENTS

_____
_____
_____
_____
_____
_____

APPOINTMENTS: _____
HEALTH CONCERNS: _____
PLANS FOR TOMORROW:_____
PAIN LEVEL: _____HAPPINESS LEVEL:_____ALERTNESS LEVEL: _____
SUPPLIES NEEDED SOON:_____
MEDICATION TAKEN:_____

NOTES

_____
_____
_____

Activity & Caregiving Notes for _____ Date:_____

TOILETING

TIME							
U							
BM							

TIMES UP DURING THE NIGHT

_____ _____ _____ _____ _____

TODAY I HAD A SHOWER/WASHED MY HAIR/SPONGE BATH

Breakfast	
AM Snack	
Lunch	
PM Snack	
Dinner	
Drinks	

ACTIVITIES & OTHER COMMENTS

_____

_____

_____

_____

_____

_____

APPOINTMENTS: _____

HEALTH CONCERNS: _____

PLANS FOR TOMORROW:_____

PAIN LEVEL: _____HAPPINESS LEVEL:_____ALERTNESS LEVEL: _____

SUPPLIES NEEDED SOON:_____

MEDICATION TAKEN:_____

NOTES

_____

_____

_____

Activity & Caregiving Notes for _____ Date:_____

TOILETING

TIME							
U							
BM							

TIMES UP DURING THE NIGHT

_____   _____   _____   _____   _____

TODAY I HAD A SHOWER/WASHED MY HAIR/SPONGE BATH

Breakfast	
AM Snack	
Lunch	
PM Snack	
Dinner	
Drinks	

ACTIVITIES & OTHER COMMENTS

_____
_____
_____
_____
_____
_____

APPOINTMENTS: _____

HEALTH CONCERNS: _____

PLANS FOR TOMORROW: _____

PAIN LEVEL: _____HAPPINESS LEVEL:_____ALERTNESS LEVEL: _____

SUPPLIES NEEDED SOON:_____

MEDICATION TAKEN:_____

NOTES

_____
_____
_____

Activity & Caregiving Notes for _____ Date:_____

TOILETING

TIME							
U							
BM							

TIMES UP DURING THE NIGHT

_____ _____ _____ _____ _____

TODAY I HAD A SHOWER/WASHED MY HAIR/SPONGE BATH

Breakfast	
AM Snack	
Lunch	
PM Snack	
Dinner	
Drinks	

ACTIVITIES & OTHER COMMENTS

_____
_____
_____
_____
_____
_____

APPOINTMENTS: _____

HEALTH CONCERNS: _____

PLANS FOR TOMORROW: _____

PAIN LEVEL: _____HAPPINESS LEVEL:_____ALERTNESS LEVEL: _____

SUPPLIES NEEDED SOON:_____

MEDICATION TAKEN:_____

NOTES

_____
_____
_____

Activity & Caregiving Notes for _____ Date:_____

TOILETING

TIME							
U							
BM							

TIMES UP DURING THE NIGHT

_____   _____   _____   _____   _____

TODAY I HAD A SHOWER/WASHED MY HAIR/SPONGE BATH

Breakfast	
AM Snack	
Lunch	
PM Snack	
Dinner	
Drinks	

ACTIVITIES & OTHER COMMENTS

_____
_____
_____
_____
_____
_____

APPOINTMENTS: _____
HEALTH CONCERNS: _____
PLANS FOR TOMORROW: _____
PAIN LEVEL: _____ HAPPINESS LEVEL:_____ALERTNESS LEVEL: _____
SUPPLIES NEEDED SOON: _____
MEDICATION TAKEN:_____

NOTES

_____
_____
_____

Activity & Caregiving Notes for _____ Date:_____

TOILETING

TIME							
U							
BM							

TIMES UP DURING THE NIGHT

_____ _____ _____ _____ _____

TODAY I HAD A SHOWER/WASHED MY HAIR/SPONGE BATH

Breakfast	
AM Snack	
Lunch	
PM Snack	
Dinner	
Drinks	

ACTIVITIES & OTHER COMMENTS

_____

_____

_____

_____

_____

_____

APPOINTMENTS: _____

HEALTH CONCERNS: _____

PLANS FOR TOMORROW: _____

PAIN LEVEL: _____ HAPPINESS LEVEL:_____ ALERTNESS LEVEL: _____

SUPPLIES NEEDED SOON:_____

MEDICATION TAKEN:_____

NOTES

_____

_____

_____

Activity & Caregiving Notes for _____ Date:_____

TOILETING

TIME							
U							
BM							

TIMES UP DURING THE NIGHT

_____ _____ _____ _____ _____

TODAY I HAD A SHOWER/WASHED MY HAIR/SPONGE BATH

Breakfast	
AM Snack	
Lunch	
PM Snack	
Dinner	
Drinks	

ACTIVITIES & OTHER COMMENTS

_____
_____
_____
_____
_____
_____

APPOINTMENTS: _____
HEALTH CONCERNS: _____
PLANS FOR TOMORROW:_____
PAIN LEVEL: _____HAPPINESS LEVEL:_____ALERTNESS LEVEL: _____
SUPPLIES NEEDED SOON:_____
MEDICATION TAKEN:_____

NOTES

_____
_____
_____

Activity & Caregiving Notes for _____ Date:_____

TOILETING

TIME								
U								
BM								

TIMES UP DURING THE NIGHT

_____   _____   _____   _____   _____

TODAY I HAD A SHOWER/WASHED MY HAIR/SPONGE BATH

Breakfast	
AM Snack	
Lunch	
PM Snack	
Dinner	
Drinks	

ACTIVITIES & OTHER COMMENTS

_____
_____
_____
_____
_____
_____
_____

APPOINTMENTS: _____

HEALTH CONCERNS: _____

PLANS FOR TOMORROW: _____

PAIN LEVEL: _____HAPPINESS LEVEL:_____ALERTNESS LEVEL: _____

SUPPLIES NEEDED SOON: _____

MEDICATION TAKEN: _____

NOTES

_____
_____
_____

Activity & Caregiving Notes for _____ Date:_____

TOILETING

TIME							
U							
BM							

TIMES UP DURING THE NIGHT

_____   _____   _____   _____   _____

TODAY I HAD A SHOWER/WASHED MY HAIR/SPONGE BATH

Breakfast	
AM Snack	
Lunch	
PM Snack	
Dinner	
Drinks	

ACTIVITIES & OTHER COMMENTS

_____
_____
_____
_____
_____
_____

APPOINTMENTS: _____

HEALTH CONCERNS:_____

PLANS FOR TOMORROW:_____

PAIN LEVEL: _____HAPPINESS LEVEL:_____ALERTNESS LEVEL: _____

SUPPLIES NEEDED SOON:_____

MEDICATION TAKEN:_____

NOTES

_____
_____
_____

Activity & Caregiving Notes for _____ Date:_____

TOILETING

TIME								
U								
BM								

TIMES UP DURING THE NIGHT

_____   _____   _____   _____   _____

TODAY I HAD A SHOWER/WASHED MY HAIR/SPONGE BATH

Breakfast	
AM Snack	
Lunch	
PM Snack	
Dinner	
Drinks	

ACTIVITIES & OTHER COMMENTS

_____

_____

_____

_____

_____

_____

APPOINTMENTS: _____

HEALTH CONCERNS: _____

PLANS FOR TOMORROW: _____

PAIN LEVEL: _____HAPPINESS LEVEL:_____ALERTNESS LEVEL: _____

SUPPLIES NEEDED SOON:_____

MEDICATION TAKEN:_____

NOTES

_____

_____

_____

Activity & Caregiving Notes for _____ Date:_____

TOILETING

TIME								
U								
BM								

TIMES UP DURING THE NIGHT

_____ _____ _____ _____ _____

TODAY I HAD A SHOWER/WASHED MY HAIR/SPONGE BATH

Breakfast	
AM Snack	
Lunch	
PM Snack	
Dinner	
Drinks	

ACTIVITIES & OTHER COMMENTS

_____

_____

_____

_____

_____

_____

APPOINTMENTS: _____

HEALTH CONCERNS: _____

PLANS FOR TOMORROW: _____

PAIN LEVEL: _____HAPPINESS LEVEL:_____ALERTNESS LEVEL: _____

SUPPLIES NEEDED SOON:_____

MEDICATION TAKEN:_____

NOTES

_____

_____

_____

Activity & Caregiving Notes for _____ Date:_____

TOILETING

TIME							
U							
BM							

TIMES UP DURING THE NIGHT

_____   _____   _____   _____   _____

TODAY I HAD A SHOWER/WASHED MY HAIR/SPONGE BATH

Breakfast	
AM Snack	
Lunch	
PM Snack	
Dinner	
Drinks	

ACTIVITIES & OTHER COMMENTS

_____
_____
_____
_____
_____
_____
_____

APPOINTMENTS: _____

HEALTH CONCERNS: _____

PLANS FOR TOMORROW: _____

PAIN LEVEL: _____HAPPINESS LEVEL:_____ALERTNESS LEVEL: _____

SUPPLIES NEEDED SOON:_____

MEDICATION TAKEN:_____

NOTES

_____
_____
_____

Activity & Caregiving Notes for _____ Date:_____

TOILETING

TIME							
U							
BM							

TIMES UP DURING THE NIGHT

_____   _____   _____   _____   _____

TODAY I HAD A SHOWER/WASHED MY HAIR/SPONGE BATH

Breakfast	
AM Snack	
Lunch	
PM Snack	
Dinner	
Drinks	

ACTIVITIES & OTHER COMMENTS

_____

_____

_____

_____

_____

_____

_____

APPOINTMENTS: _____

HEALTH CONCERNS: _____

PLANS FOR TOMORROW: _____

PAIN LEVEL: _____HAPPINESS LEVEL:_____ALERTNESS LEVEL: _____

SUPPLIES NEEDED SOON: _____

MEDICATION TAKEN:_____

NOTES

_____

_____

_____

Activity & Caregiving Notes for _____ Date:_____

TOILETING

TIME							
U							
BM							

TIMES UP DURING THE NIGHT

_____   _____   _____   _____   _____

TODAY I HAD A SHOWER/WASHED MY HAIR/SPONGE BATH

Breakfast	
AM Snack	
Lunch	
PM Snack	
Dinner	
Drinks	

ACTIVITIES & OTHER COMMENTS

_____

_____

_____

_____

_____

_____

APPOINTMENTS: _____

HEALTH CONCERNS: _____

PLANS FOR TOMORROW: _____

PAIN LEVEL: _____ HAPPINESS LEVEL:_____ ALERTNESS LEVEL: _____

SUPPLIES NEEDED SOON:_____

MEDICATION TAKEN:_____

NOTES

_____

_____

_____

Activity & Caregiving Notes for _____ Date:_____

TOILETING

TIME							
U							
BM							

TIMES UP DURING THE NIGHT

_____ _____ _____ _____ _____

TODAY I HAD A SHOWER/WASHED MY HAIR/SPONGE BATH

Breakfast	
AM Snack	
Lunch	
PM Snack	
Dinner	
Drinks	

ACTIVITIES & OTHER COMMENTS

_____
_____
_____
_____
_____
_____

APPOINTMENTS: _____
HEALTH CONCERNS:_____
PLANS FOR TOMORROW:_____
PAIN LEVEL: _____HAPPINESS LEVEL:_____ALERTNESS LEVEL: _____
SUPPLIES NEEDED SOON:_____
MEDICATION TAKEN:_____

NOTES

_____
_____
_____

Activity & Caregiving Notes for _____ Date:_____

TOILETING

TIME							
U							
BM							

TIMES UP DURING THE NIGHT

_____ _____ _____ _____ _____

TODAY I HAD A SHOWER/WASHED MY HAIR/SPONGE BATH

Breakfast	
AM Snack	
Lunch	
PM Snack	
Dinner	
Drinks	

ACTIVITIES & OTHER COMMENTS

_____
_____
_____
_____
_____
_____

APPOINTMENTS: _____

HEALTH CONCERNS: _____

PLANS FOR TOMORROW: _____

PAIN LEVEL: _____HAPPINESS LEVEL:_____ALERTNESS LEVEL: _____

SUPPLIES NEEDED SOON: _____

MEDICATION TAKEN:_____

NOTES

_____
_____
_____

Activity & Caregiving Notes for _____ Date:_____

TOILETING

TIME								
U								
BM								

TIMES UP DURING THE NIGHT

_____ _____ _____ _____ _____

TODAY I HAD A SHOWER/WASHED MY HAIR/SPONGE BATH

Breakfast	
AM Snack	
Lunch	
PM Snack	
Dinner	
Drinks	

ACTIVITIES & OTHER COMMENTS

_____
_____
_____
_____
_____
_____

APPOINTMENTS: _____

HEALTH CONCERNS:_____

PLANS FOR TOMORROW:_____

PAIN LEVEL: _____HAPPINESS LEVEL:_____ALERTNESS LEVEL: _____

SUPPLIES NEEDED SOON:_____

MEDICATION TAKEN:_____

NOTES

_____
_____
_____

Activity & Caregiving Notes for _____ Date:_____

TOILETING

TIME							
U							
BM							

TIMES UP DURING THE NIGHT

_____ _____ _____ _____ _____

TODAY I HAD A SHOWER/WASHED MY HAIR/SPONGE BATH

Breakfast	
AM Snack	
Lunch	
PM Snack	
Dinner	
Drinks	

ACTIVITIES & OTHER COMMENTS

_____
_____
_____
_____
_____
_____
_____

APPOINTMENTS: _____

HEALTH CONCERNS: _____

PLANS FOR TOMORROW: _____

PAIN LEVEL: _____ HAPPINESS LEVEL:_____ ALERTNESS LEVEL: _____

SUPPLIES NEEDED SOON:_____

MEDICATION TAKEN:_____

NOTES

_____
_____
_____

Activity & Caregiving Notes for _____ Date:_____

TOILETING

TIME							
U							
BM							

TIMES UP DURING THE NIGHT

_____   _____   _____   _____   _____

TODAY I HAD A SHOWER/WASHED MY HAIR/SPONGE BATH

Breakfast	
AM Snack	
Lunch	
PM Snack	
Dinner	
Drinks	

ACTIVITIES & OTHER COMMENTS

_____
_____
_____
_____
_____
_____

APPOINTMENTS: _____
HEALTH CONCERNS: _____
PLANS FOR TOMORROW:_____
PAIN LEVEL: _____HAPPINESS LEVEL:_____ALERTNESS LEVEL: _____
SUPPLIES NEEDED SOON: _____
MEDICATION TAKEN:_____

NOTES

_____
_____
_____

Activity & Caregiving Notes for _____ Date:_____

TOILETING

TIME							
U							
BM							

TIMES UP DURING THE NIGHT

_____   _____   _____   _____   _____

TODAY I HAD A SHOWER/WASHED MY HAIR/SPONGE BATH

Breakfast	
AM Snack	
Lunch	
PM Snack	
Dinner	
Drinks	

ACTIVITIES & OTHER COMMENTS

_____
_____
_____
_____
_____
_____

APPOINTMENTS: _____

HEALTH CONCERNS: _____

PLANS FOR TOMORROW: _____

PAIN LEVEL: _____HAPPINESS LEVEL:_____ALERTNESS LEVEL: _____

SUPPLIES NEEDED SOON:_____

MEDICATION TAKEN:_____

NOTES

_____
_____
_____

Activity & Caregiving Notes for _____ Date:_____

TOILETING

TIME							
U							
BM							

TIMES UP DURING THE NIGHT

_____ _____ _____ _____ _____

TODAY I HAD A SHOWER/WASHED MY HAIR/SPONGE BATH

Breakfast	
AM Snack	
Lunch	
PM Snack	
Dinner	
Drinks	

ACTIVITIES & OTHER COMMENTS

_____
_____
_____
_____
_____
_____

APPOINTMENTS: _____

HEALTH CONCERNS: _____

PLANS FOR TOMORROW: _____

PAIN LEVEL: _____HAPPINESS LEVEL:_____ALERTNESS LEVEL: _____

SUPPLIES NEEDED SOON: _____

MEDICATION TAKEN:_____

NOTES

_____
_____
_____

Activity & Caregiving Notes for _____ Date:_____

TOILETING

TIME							
U							
BM							

TIMES UP DURING THE NIGHT

_____   _____   _____   _____   _____

TODAY I HAD A SHOWER/WASHED MY HAIR/SPONGE BATH

Breakfast	
AM Snack	
Lunch	
PM Snack	
Dinner	
Drinks	

ACTIVITIES & OTHER COMMENTS

_____
_____
_____
_____
_____
_____

APPOINTMENTS: _____

HEALTH CONCERNS: _____

PLANS FOR TOMORROW: _____

PAIN LEVEL: _____ HAPPINESS LEVEL:_____ALERTNESS LEVEL: _____

SUPPLIES NEEDED SOON:_____

MEDICATION TAKEN:_____

NOTES

_____
_____
_____

Activity & Caregiving Notes for _____ Date:_____

TOILETING

TIME							
U							
BM							

TIMES UP DURING THE NIGHT

_____   _____   _____   _____   _____

TODAY I HAD A SHOWER/WASHED MY HAIR/SPONGE BATH

Breakfast	
AM Snack	
Lunch	
PM Snack	
Dinner	
Drinks	

ACTIVITIES & OTHER COMMENTS

_____
_____
_____
_____
_____
_____

APPOINTMENTS: _____

HEALTH CONCERNS: _____

PLANS FOR TOMORROW: _____

PAIN LEVEL: _____HAPPINESS LEVEL:_____ALERTNESS LEVEL: _____

SUPPLIES NEEDED SOON: _____

MEDICATION TAKEN:_____

NOTES

_____
_____
_____

Activity & Caregiving Notes for _____ Date:_____

TOILETING

TIME							
U							
BM							

TIMES UP DURING THE NIGHT

_____ _____ _____ _____ _____

TODAY I HAD A SHOWER/WASHED MY HAIR/SPONGE BATH

Breakfast	
AM Snack	
Lunch	
PM Snack	
Dinner	
Drinks	

ACTIVITIES & OTHER COMMENTS

_____
_____
_____
_____
_____
_____

APPOINTMENTS: _____
HEALTH CONCERNS: _____
PLANS FOR TOMORROW: _____
PAIN LEVEL: _____ HAPPINESS LEVEL:_____ALERTNESS LEVEL: _____
SUPPLIES NEEDED SOON: _____
MEDICATION TAKEN:_____

NOTES

_____
_____
_____

Activity & Caregiving Notes for _____ Date:_____

TOILETING

TIME							
U							
BM							

TIMES UP DURING THE NIGHT

_____   _____   _____   _____   _____

TODAY I HAD A SHOWER/WASHED MY HAIR/SPONGE BATH

Breakfast	
AM Snack	
Lunch	
PM Snack	
Dinner	
Drinks	

ACTIVITIES & OTHER COMMENTS

_____

_____

_____

_____

_____

_____

APPOINTMENTS: _____

HEALTH CONCERNS: _____

PLANS FOR TOMORROW: _____

PAIN LEVEL: _____HAPPINESS LEVEL:_____ALERTNESS LEVEL: _____

SUPPLIES NEEDED SOON: _____

MEDICATION TAKEN:_____

NOTES

_____

_____

_____

Activity & Caregiving Notes for _____ Date:_____

TOILETING

TIME								
U								
BM								

TIMES UP DURING THE NIGHT

_____   _____   _____   _____   _____

TODAY I HAD A SHOWER/WASHED MY HAIR/SPONGE BATH

Breakfast	
AM Snack	
Lunch	
PM Snack	
Dinner	
Drinks	

ACTIVITIES & OTHER COMMENTS

_____

_____

_____

_____

_____

_____

APPOINTMENTS: _____

HEALTH CONCERNS: _____

PLANS FOR TOMORROW: _____

PAIN LEVEL: _____ HAPPINESS LEVEL:_____ ALERTNESS LEVEL: _____

SUPPLIES NEEDED SOON: _____

MEDICATION TAKEN: _____

NOTES

_____

_____

_____

Activity & Caregiving Notes for _____ Date:_____

TOILETING

TIME							
U							
BM							

TIMES UP DURING THE NIGHT

_____ _____ _____ _____ _____

TODAY I HAD A SHOWER/WASHED MY HAIR/SPONGE BATH

Breakfast	
AM Snack	
Lunch	
PM Snack	
Dinner	
Drinks	

ACTIVITIES & OTHER COMMENTS

_____
_____
_____
_____
_____
_____

APPOINTMENTS: _____

HEALTH CONCERNS: _____

PLANS FOR TOMORROW: _____

PAIN LEVEL: _____ HAPPINESS LEVEL:_____ ALERTNESS LEVEL: _____

SUPPLIES NEEDED SOON:_____

MEDICATION TAKEN:_____

NOTES

_____
_____
_____

Activity & Caregiving Notes for _____ Date:_____

TOILETING

TIME								
U								
BM								

TIMES UP DURING THE NIGHT

_____ _____ _____ _____ _____

TODAY I HAD A SHOWER/WASHED MY HAIR/SPONGE BATH

Breakfast	
AM Snack	
Lunch	
PM Snack	
Dinner	
Drinks	

ACTIVITIES & OTHER COMMENTS

_____

_____

_____

_____

_____

_____

APPOINTMENTS: _____

HEALTH CONCERNS: _____

PLANS FOR TOMORROW: _____

PAIN LEVEL: _____HAPPINESS LEVEL:_____ALERTNESS LEVEL: _____

SUPPLIES NEEDED SOON: _____

MEDICATION TAKEN:_____

NOTES

_____

_____

_____

Activity & Caregiving Notes for _____ Date:_____

TOILETING

TIME							
U							
BM							

TIMES UP DURING THE NIGHT

_____   _____   _____   _____   _____

TODAY I HAD A SHOWER/WASHED MY HAIR/SPONGE BATH

Breakfast	
AM Snack	
Lunch	
PM Snack	
Dinner	
Drinks	

ACTIVITIES & OTHER COMMENTS

_____
_____
_____
_____
_____
_____

APPOINTMENTS: _____

HEALTH CONCERNS: _____

PLANS FOR TOMORROW: _____

PAIN LEVEL: _____HAPPINESS LEVEL:_____ALERTNESS LEVEL: _____

SUPPLIES NEEDED SOON:_____

MEDICATION TAKEN:_____

NOTES

_____
_____
_____

Activity & Caregiving Notes for _____ Date:_____

TOILETING

TIME							
U							
BM							

TIMES UP DURING THE NIGHT

_____   _____   _____   _____   _____

TODAY I HAD A SHOWER/WASHED MY HAIR/SPONGE BATH

Breakfast	
AM Snack	
Lunch	
PM Snack	
Dinner	
Drinks	

ACTIVITIES & OTHER COMMENTS

_____
_____
_____
_____
_____
_____

APPOINTMENTS: _____
HEALTH CONCERNS: _____
PLANS FOR TOMORROW: _____
PAIN LEVEL: _____HAPPINESS LEVEL:_____ALERTNESS LEVEL: _____
SUPPLIES NEEDED SOON:_____
MEDICATION TAKEN:_____

NOTES

_____
_____
_____

Activity & Caregiving Notes for _____ Date:_____

TOILETING

TIME								
U								
BM								

TIMES UP DURING THE NIGHT

_____ _____ _____ _____ _____

TODAY I HAD A SHOWER/WASHED MY HAIR/SPONGE BATH

Breakfast	
AM Snack	
Lunch	
PM Snack	
Dinner	
Drinks	

ACTIVITIES & OTHER COMMENTS

_____

_____

_____

_____

_____

_____

APPOINTMENTS: _____

HEALTH CONCERNS: _____

PLANS FOR TOMORROW:_____

PAIN LEVEL: _____HAPPINESS LEVEL:_____ALERTNESS LEVEL: _____

SUPPLIES NEEDED SOON:_____

MEDICATION TAKEN:_____

NOTES

_____

_____

_____

Activity & Caregiving Notes for _____ Date:_____

TOILETING

TIME							
U							
BM							

TIMES UP DURING THE NIGHT

_____ _____ _____ _____ _____

TODAY I HAD A SHOWER/WASHED MY HAIR/SPONGE BATH

Breakfast	
AM Snack	
Lunch	
PM Snack	
Dinner	
Drinks	

ACTIVITIES & OTHER COMMENTS

_____
_____
_____
_____
_____
_____

APPOINTMENTS: _____
HEALTH CONCERNS: _____
PLANS FOR TOMORROW: _____
PAIN LEVEL: _____ HAPPINESS LEVEL:_____ ALERTNESS LEVEL: _____
SUPPLIES NEEDED SOON: _____
MEDICATION TAKEN:_____

NOTES

_____
_____
_____

Activity & Caregiving Notes for _____ Date:_____

TOILETING

TIME							
U							
BM							

TIMES UP DURING THE NIGHT

_____   _____   _____   _____   _____

TODAY I HAD A SHOWER/WASHED MY HAIR/SPONGE BATH

Breakfast	
AM Snack	
Lunch	
PM Snack	
Dinner	
Drinks	

ACTIVITIES & OTHER COMMENTS

_____

_____

_____

_____

_____

_____

APPOINTMENTS: _____

HEALTH CONCERNS: _____

PLANS FOR TOMORROW: _____

PAIN LEVEL: _____HAPPINESS LEVEL:_____ALERTNESS LEVEL: _____

SUPPLIES NEEDED SOON: _____

MEDICATION TAKEN:_____

NOTES

_____

_____

_____

Activity & Caregiving Notes for _____ Date:_____

TOILETING

TIME							
U							
BM							

TIMES UP DURING THE NIGHT

_____ _____ _____ _____ _____

TODAY I HAD A SHOWER/WASHED MY HAIR/SPONGE BATH

Breakfast	
AM Snack	
Lunch	
PM Snack	
Dinner	
Drinks	

ACTIVITIES & OTHER COMMENTS

_____

_____

_____

_____

_____

_____

APPOINTMENTS: _____

HEALTH CONCERNS: _____

PLANS FOR TOMORROW: _____

PAIN LEVEL: _____ HAPPINESS LEVEL:_____ ALERTNESS LEVEL: _____

SUPPLIES NEEDED SOON: _____

MEDICATION TAKEN: _____

NOTES

_____

_____

_____

Activity & Caregiving Notes for _____ Date:_____

TOILETING

TIME							
U							
BM							

TIMES UP DURING THE NIGHT

_____ _____ _____ _____ _____

TODAY I HAD A SHOWER/WASHED MY HAIR/SPONGE BATH

Breakfast	
AM Snack	
Lunch	
PM Snack	
Dinner	
Drinks	

ACTIVITIES & OTHER COMMENTS

_____
_____
_____
_____
_____
_____

APPOINTMENTS: _____
HEALTH CONCERNS: _____
PLANS FOR TOMORROW: _____
PAIN LEVEL: _____HAPPINESS LEVEL:_____ALERTNESS LEVEL: _____
SUPPLIES NEEDED SOON: _____
MEDICATION TAKEN:_____

NOTES

_____
_____
_____

Activity & Caregiving Notes for _____ Date:_____

TOILETING

TIME							
U							
BM							

TIMES UP DURING THE NIGHT

_____   _____   _____   _____   _____

TODAY I HAD A SHOWER/WASHED MY HAIR/SPONGE BATH

Breakfast	
AM Snack	
Lunch	
PM Snack	
Dinner	
Drinks	

ACTIVITIES & OTHER COMMENTS

_____
_____
_____
_____
_____
_____

APPOINTMENTS: _____

HEALTH CONCERNS: _____

PLANS FOR TOMORROW: _____

PAIN LEVEL: _____ HAPPINESS LEVEL:_____ ALERTNESS LEVEL: _____

SUPPLIES NEEDED SOON:_____

MEDICATION TAKEN:_____

NOTES

_____
_____
_____

Activity & Caregiving Notes for _____ Date:_____

TOILETING

TIME							
U							
BM							

TIMES UP DURING THE NIGHT

_____ _____ _____ _____ _____

TODAY I HAD A SHOWER/WASHED MY HAIR/SPONGE BATH

Breakfast	
AM Snack	
Lunch	
PM Snack	
Dinner	
Drinks	

ACTIVITIES & OTHER COMMENTS

_____
_____
_____
_____
_____
_____

APPOINTMENTS: _____

HEALTH CONCERNS: _____

PLANS FOR TOMORROW: _____

PAIN LEVEL: _____HAPPINESS LEVEL:_____ALERTNESS LEVEL: _____

SUPPLIES NEEDED SOON: _____

MEDICATION TAKEN:_____

NOTES

_____
_____
_____

Activity & Caregiving Notes for _____ Date:_____

TOILETING

TIME							
U							
BM							

TIMES UP DURING THE NIGHT

_____   _____   _____   _____   _____

TODAY I HAD A SHOWER/WASHED MY HAIR/SPONGE BATH

Breakfast	
AM Snack	
Lunch	
PM Snack	
Dinner	
Drinks	

ACTIVITIES & OTHER COMMENTS

_____
_____
_____
_____
_____
_____

APPOINTMENTS: _____

HEALTH CONCERNS: _____

PLANS FOR TOMORROW: _____

PAIN LEVEL: _____ HAPPINESS LEVEL:_____ ALERTNESS LEVEL: _____

SUPPLIES NEEDED SOON: _____

MEDICATION TAKEN: _____

NOTES

_____
_____
_____

Made in United States
North Haven, CT
23 January 2023